Healthy Slow Cooker Cookbook for Beginners

The Best Recipes for Living and Eating Well.

By Jaclyn Mirrel

Sommario

Introduction

We understand you are constantly trying to find much easier means to prepare your meals. We likewise understand you are probably sick and tired of spending long hrs in the kitchen cooking

with a lot of frying pans and also pots. Well, currently your search mores than! We located the excellent kitchen area device you can use from now on! We are discussing the Slow stove!

These fantastic pots permit you to prepare several of the best dishes ever with minimal initiative Slow-moving stoves cook your dishes less complicated and a whole lot much healthier! You do not need to be a specialist in the kitchen to cook several of the most tasty, flavorful, textured and abundant meals!

All you need is your Slow stove as well as the appropriate active ingredients!
This wonderful cookbook you are about to discover will certainly show you exactly how to cook the best slow cooked meals. It will certainly reveal you that you can make some outstanding

breakfasts, lunch meals, side meals, poultry, meat and also fish dishes.

Ultimately yet significantly, this cookbook gives you some straightforward and sweet treats.

Chili Eggs Mix

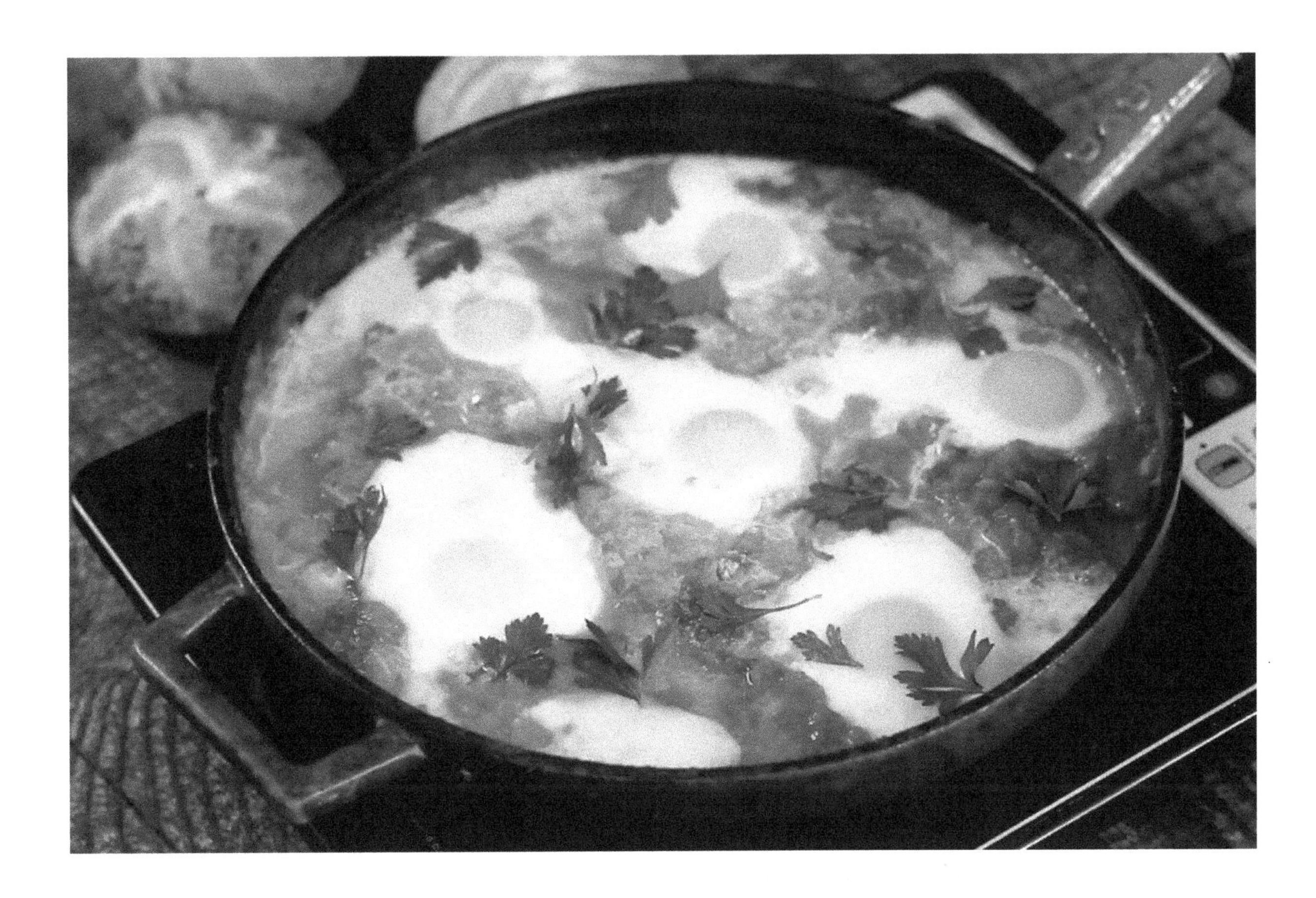

Preparation time: 10 minutes

Cooking time: 3 hours

Servings: 2

Ingredients:

- Cooking spray
- 3 spring onions, chopped
- 2 tablespoons sun dried tomatoes, chopped
- 1 ounce canned and roasted green chili pepper, chopped
- ½ teaspoon rosemary, dried
- Salt and black pepper to the taste
- 3 ounces cheddar cheese, shredded
- 4 eggs, whisked
- ¼ cup heavy cream
- 1 tablespoon chives, chopped

Directions:

1. Grease your slow cooker with cooking spray and mix the eggs with the chili peppers and the other ingredients except the cheese.

2. Toss everything into the pot, sprinkle the cheese on top, put the lid on and cook on High for 3 hours.
3. Divide between plates and serve.

Nutrition: calories 224, fat 4, fiber 7, carbs 18, protein 11

Cheesy Eggs

Preparation time: 10 minutes

Cooking time: 3 hours

Servings: 2

Ingredients:

- 4 eggs, whisked
- ¼ cup spring onions, chopped
- 1 tablespoon oregano, chopped
- 1 cup milk
- 2 ounces feta cheese, crumbled
- A pinch of salt and black pepper
- Cooking spray

Directions:

1. In a bowl, combine the eggs with the spring onions and the other ingredients except the cooking spray and whisk.

2. Grease your slow cooker with cooking spray, add eggs mix, stir , put the lid on and cook on Low for 3 hours.

3. Divide between plates and serve for breakfast.

Nutrition: calories 214, fat 4, fiber 7, carbs 18, protein 5

Creamy Strawberries Oatmeal

Preparation time: 10 minutes

Cooking time: 8 hours

Servings: 8

Ingredients:

- 6 cups water
- 2 cups milk
- 2 cups steel cut oats
- 1 cup Greek yogurt
- 1 teaspoon cinnamon powder
- 2 cups strawberries, halved
- 1 teaspoon vanilla extract

Directions:

1. In your Slow cooker, mix water with milk, oats, yogurt, cinnamon, strawberries and vanilla, toss, cover and cook on Low for 8 hours.

2. Divide into bowls and serve for breakfast.

Nutrition: calories 200, fat 4, fiber 6, carbs 8, protein 4

Tomato and Zucchini Eggs Mix

Preparation time: 10 minutes

Cooking time: 3 hours

Servings: 2

Ingredients:

- Cooking spray
- 4 eggs, whisked
- 2 spring onions, chopped
- 1 tablespoon basil, chopped
- ½ teaspoon turmeric powder
- ½ cup tomatoes, cubed
- 1 zucchini, grated
- ¼ teaspoon sweet paprika

- A pinch of salt and black pepper
- 1 tablespoon parsley, chopped
- 2 tablespoons parmesan, grated

Directions:

1. Grease your slow cooker with cooking spray, add the eggs mixed with the zucchini, tomatoes and the other ingredients except the cheese and stir well.
2. Sprinkle the cheese, put the lid on and cook on High for 3 hours.
3. Divide between plates and serve for breakfast right away.

Nutrition: calories 261, fat 5, fiber 7, carbs 19, protein 6

Breakfast Potatoes

Preparation time: 10 minutes

Cooking time: 4 hours

Servings: 8

Ingredients:

- 3 potatoes, peeled and cubed
- 1 green bell pepper, chopped
- 1 red bell pepper, chopped
- 1 yellow onion, chopped
- 12 ounces smoked chicken sausage, sliced
- 1 and ½ cups cheddar cheese, shredded
- ¼ teaspoon oregano, dried
- ½ cup sour cream

- ¼ teaspoon basil, dried
- 10 ounces cream of chicken soup
- 2 tablespoons parsley, chopped
- Salt and black pepper to the taste

Directions:

1. In your Slow cooker, mix potatoes with red bell pepper, green bell pepper, sausage, onion, oregano, basil, cheese, salt, pepper and cream of chicken, cover and cook on Low for 4 hours.
2. Add parsley, divide between plates and serve for breakfast.

Nutrition: calories 320, fat 5, fiber 7, carbs 10, protein 5

Chocolate Breakfast Bread

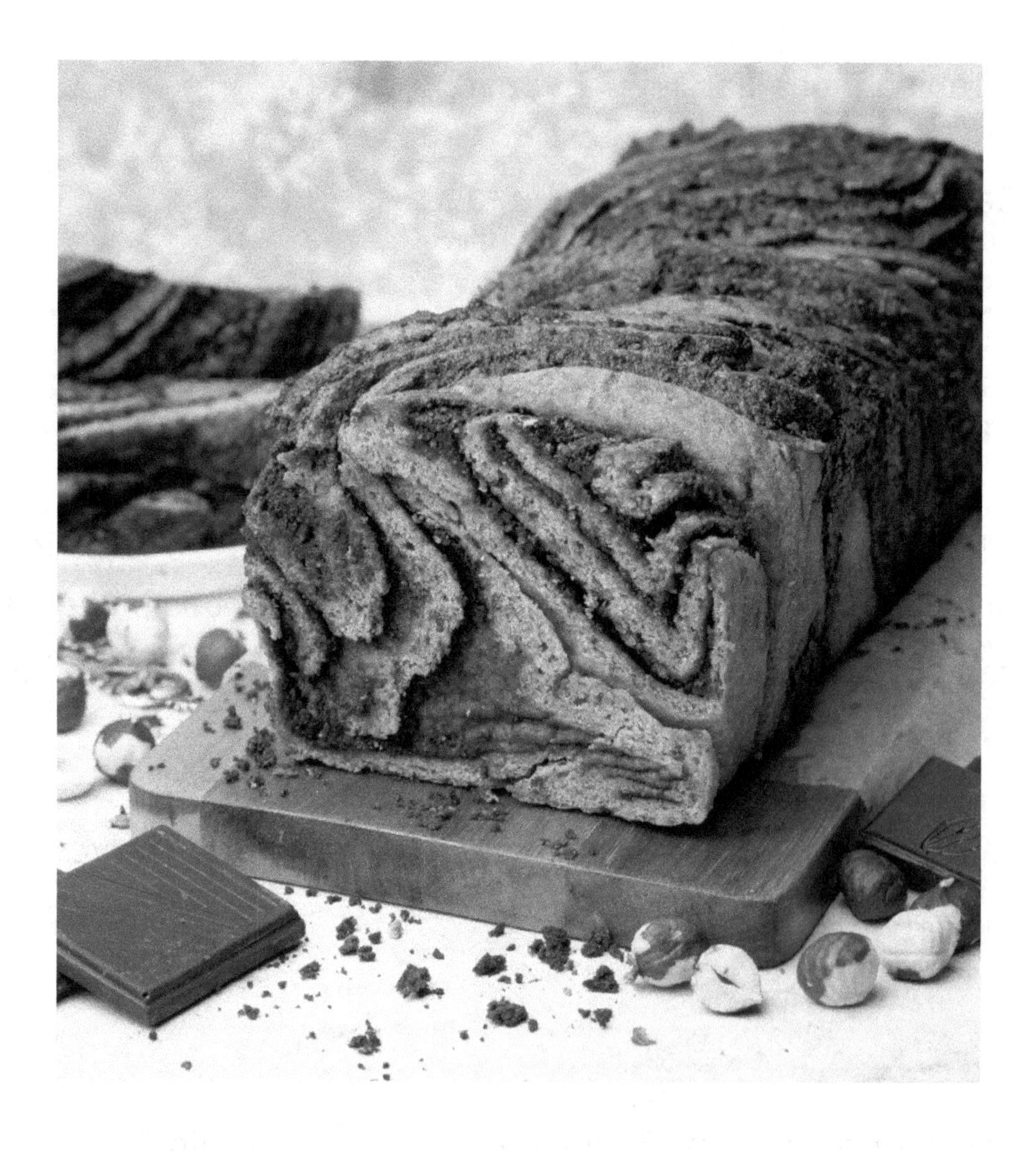

Preparation time: 10 minutes

Cooking time: 3 hours

Servings: 2

Ingredients:

- Cooking spray
- 1 cup almond flour
- ½ teaspoon baking soda
- ½ teaspoon cinnamon powder
- 1 tablespoon avocado oil
- 2 tablespoons maple syrup
- 2 eggs, whisked
- 1 tablespoon butter
- ½ tablespoon milk
- ½ teaspoon vanilla extract
- ½ cup dark chocolate, melted
- 2 tablespoons walnuts, chopped

Directions:

1. In a bowl, mix the flour with the baking soda, cinnamon, oil and the other ingredients except the cooking spray and stir well.

2. Grease a loaf pan that fits the slow cooker with the cooking spray, pour the bread batter into the pan, put the pan in the slow cooker after you've lined it with tin foil, put the lid on and cook on High for 3 hours.

3. Cool the sweet bread down, slice, divide between plates and serve for breakfast.

Nutrition: calories 200, fat 3, fiber 5, carbs 8, protein 4

Hash Brown Mix

Preparation time: 10 minutes

Cooking time: 3 hours

Servings: 6

Ingredients:

- 3 tablespoons butter
- ½ cup sour cream
- ¼ cup mushrooms, sliced
- ¼ teaspoon garlic powder
- ¼ cup yellow onion, chopped
- 1 cup milk
- 3 tablespoons flour

- 20 ounces hash browns
- Salt and black pepper to the taste
- 1 cup cheddar cheese, shredded
- Cooking spray

Directions:

1. Heat up a pan with the butter over medium-high heat, add mushrooms, onion and garlic powder, stir and cook for a few minutes.
2. Add flour and whisk well.
3. Add milk, stir really well and transfer everything to your Slow cooker greased with cooking spray.
4. Add hash browns, salt, pepper, sour cream and cheese, toss, cover and cook on High for 3 hours.
5. Divide between plates and serve for breakfast.

Nutrition: calories 262, fat 6, fiber 4, carbs 12, protein 6

Almond and Quinoa Bowls

Preparation time: 10 minutes

Cooking time: 5 hours

Servings: 2

Ingredients:

- 1 cup quinoa
- 2 cups almond milk
- 2 tablespoons butter, melted
- 2 tablespoons brown sugar
- A pinch of cinnamon powder
- A pinch of nutmeg, ground
- ¼ cup almonds, sliced
- Cooking spray

Directions:

1. Grease your slow cooker with the cooking spray, add the quinoa, milk, melted butter and the other ingredients, toss, put the lid on and cook on Low for 5 hours.

2. Divide the mix into bowls and serve for breakfast.

Nutrition: calories 211, fat 3, fiber 6, carbs 12, protein 5

Bacon and Egg Casserole

Preparation time: 10 minutes

Cooking time: 5 hours

Servings: 8

Ingredients:

- 20 ounces hash browns
- Cooking spray
- 8 ounces cheddar cheese, shredded
- 8 bacon slices, cooked and chopped
- 6 green onions, chopped
- ½ cup milk
- 12 eggs
- Salt and black pepper to the taste

- Salsa for serving

Directions:

1. Grease your Slow cooker with cooking spray, spread hash browns, cheese, bacon and green onions and toss.
2. In a bowl, mix the eggs with salt, pepper and milk and whisk really well.
3. Pour this over hash browns, cover and cook on Low for 5 hours.
4. Divide between plates and serve with salsa on top.

Nutrition: calories 300, fat 5, fiber 5, carbs 9, protein 5

Carrots Casserole

Preparation time: 10 minutes

Cooking time: 3 hours

Servings: 2

Ingredients:

- 1 teaspoon ginger, ground
- ½ pound carrots, peeled and grated
- 2 eggs, whisked
- ½ teaspoon garlic powder
- ½ teaspoon rosemary, dried
- Salt and black pepper to the taste
- 1 red onion, chopped
- 1 tablespoons parsley, chopped

- 2 garlic cloves, minced
- ½ tablespoon olive oil

Directions:

1. Grease your slow cooker with the oil and mix the carrots with the eggs, ginger and the other ingredients inside.
2. Toss, put the lid on, cook High for 3 hours, divide between plates and serve.

Nutrition: calories 218, fat 6, fiber 6, carbs 14, protein 5

Breakfast Rice Pudding

Preparation time: 10 minutes

Cooking time: 4 hours

Servings: 4

Ingredients:

- 1 cup coconut milk
- 2 cups water
- 1 cup almond milk
- ½ cup raisins
- 1 cup brown rice
- 2 teaspoons vanilla extract
- 2 tablespoons flaxseed
- 1 teaspoon cinnamon powder

- 2 tablespoons coconut sugar
- Cooking spray

Directions:

1. Grease your Slow cooker with the cooking spray, add coconut milk, water, almond milk, raisins, rice, vanilla, flaxseed and cinnamon, cover, cook on Low for 4 hours, stir, divide into bowls, sprinkle coconut sugar all over and serve.

Nutrition: calories 213, fat 3, fiber 6, carbs 10, protein 4

Cranberry Maple Oatmeal

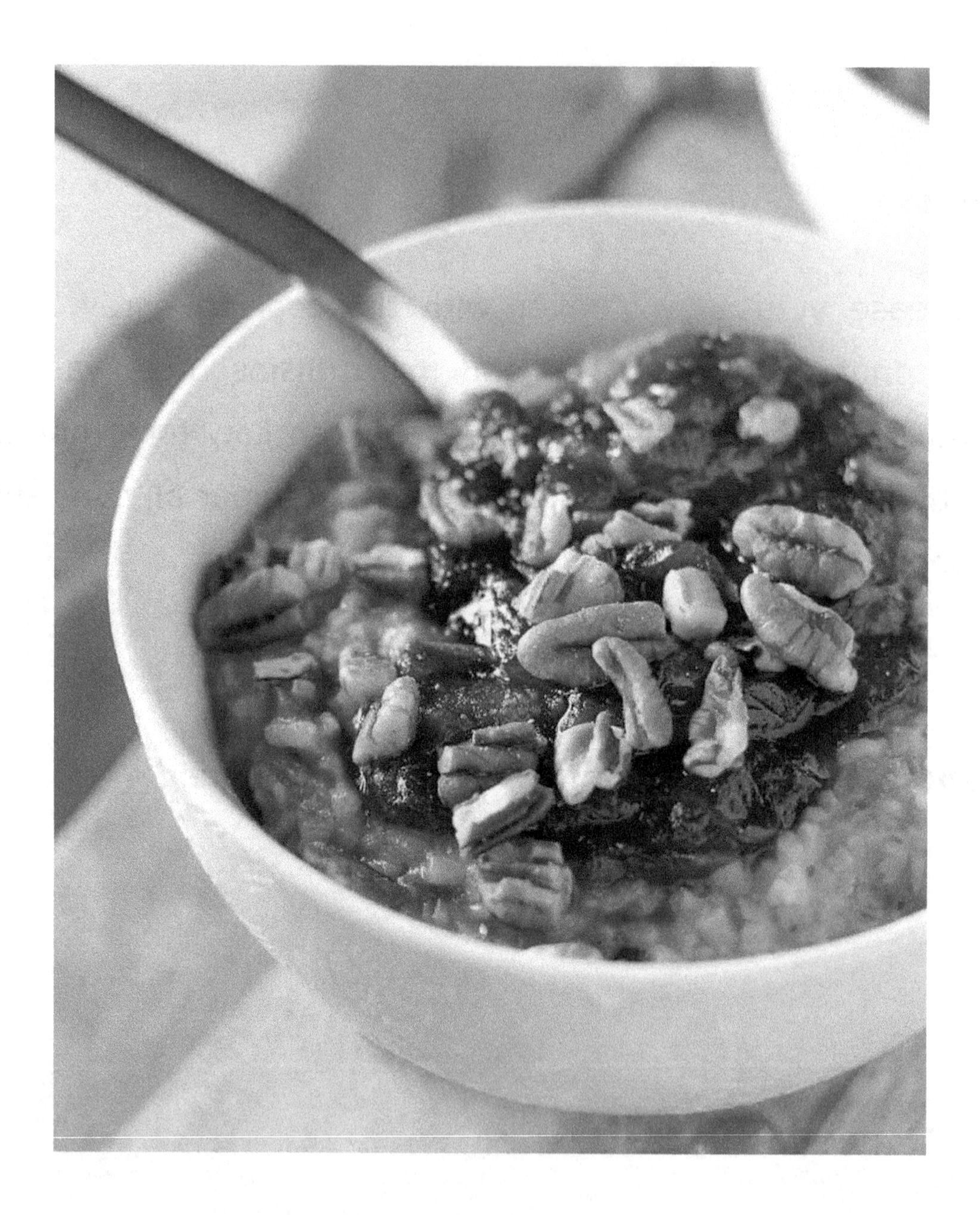

Preparation time: 10 minutes

Cooking time: 6 hours

Servings: 2

Ingredients:

- 1 cup almond milk
- ½ cup steel cut oats
- ½ cup cranberries
- ½ teaspoon vanilla extract
- 1 tablespoon maple syrup
- 1 tablespoon sugar

Directions:

1. In your slow cooker, mix the oats with the berries, milk and the other ingredients, toss, put the lid on and cook on Low for 6 hours.

2. Divide into bowls and serve for breakfast.

Nutrition: calories 200, fat 5, fiber 7, carbs 14, protein 4

Apple Breakfast Rice

Preparation time: 10 minutes

Cooking time: 7 hours

Servings: 4

Ingredients:

- 4 apples, cored, peeled and chopped
- 2 tablespoons butter
- 2 teaspoons cinnamon powder
- 1 and ½ cups brown rice
- ½ teaspoon vanilla extract
- A pinch of nutmeg, ground
- 5 cups milk

Directions:

1. Put the butter in your Slow cooker, add apples, cinnamon, rice, vanilla, nutmeg and milk, cover, cook on Low for 7 hours, stir, divide into bowls and serve for breakfast.

Nutrition: calories 214, fat 4, fiber 5, carbs 7, protein 4

Mushroom Casserole

Preparation time: 10 minutes

Cooking time: 5 hours

Servings: 2

Ingredients:

- ½ cup mozzarella, shredded
- 2 eggs, whisked
- ½ tablespoon balsamic vinegar
- ½ tablespoon olive oil
- 4 ounces baby kale
- 1 red onion, chopped
- ¼ teaspoon oregano
- ½ pound white mushrooms, sliced

- Salt and black pepper to the taste
- Cooking spray

Directions:

1. In a bowl, mix the eggs with the kale, mushrooms and the other ingredients except the cheese and cooking spray and stir well.
2. Grease your slow cooker with cooking spray, add the mushroom mix, spread, sprinkle the mozzarella all over, put the lid on and cook on Low for 5 hours.
3. Divide between plates and serve for breakfast.

Nutrition: calories 216, fat 6, fiber 8, carbs 12, protein 4

Quinoa and Banana Mix

Preparation time: 10 minutes

Cooking time: 6 hours

Servings: 8

Ingredients:

- 2 cups quinoa
- 2 bananas, mashed
- 4 cups water
- 2 cups blueberries
- 2 teaspoons vanilla extract
- 2 tablespoons maple syrup
- 1 teaspoon cinnamon powder
- Cooking spray

Directions:

1. Grease your Slow cooker with cooking spray, add quinoa, bananas, water, blueberries, vanilla, maple syrup and cinnamon, stir, cover and cook on Low for 6 hours.

2. Stir again, divide into bowls and serve for breakfast.

Nutrition: calories 200, fat 4, fiber 6, carbs 12, protein 4

Ginger Apple Bowls

Preparation time: 10 minutes

Cooking time: 6 hours

Servings: 2

Ingredients:

- 2 apples, cored, peeled and cut into medium chunks
- 1 tablespoon sugar
- 1 tablespoon ginger, grated
- 1 cup heavy cream
- ¼ teaspoon cinnamon powder
- ½ teaspoon vanilla extract
- ¼ teaspoon cardamom, ground

Directions:

1. In your slow cooker, combine the apples with the sugar, ginger and the other ingredients, toss, put the lid on and cook on Low for 6 hours.

2. Divide into bowls and serve for breakfast.

Nutrition: calories 201, fat 3, fiber 7, carbs 19, protein 4

Dates Quinoa

Preparation time: 10 minutes

Cooking time: 3 hours

Servings: 4

Ingredients:

- 1 cup quinoa
- 4 medjol dates, chopped
- 3 cups milk
- 1 apple, cored and chopped
- ¼ cup pepitas
- 2 teaspoons cinnamon powder
- 1 teaspoon vanilla extract
- ¼ teaspoon nutmeg, ground

Directions:

1. In your Slow cooker, mix quinoa with dates, milk, apple, pepitas, cinnamon, nutmeg and vanilla, stir, cover and cook on High for 3 hours.

2. Stir again, divide into bowls and serve.

Nutrition: calories 241, fat 4, fiber 4, carbs 10, protein 3

Granola Bowls

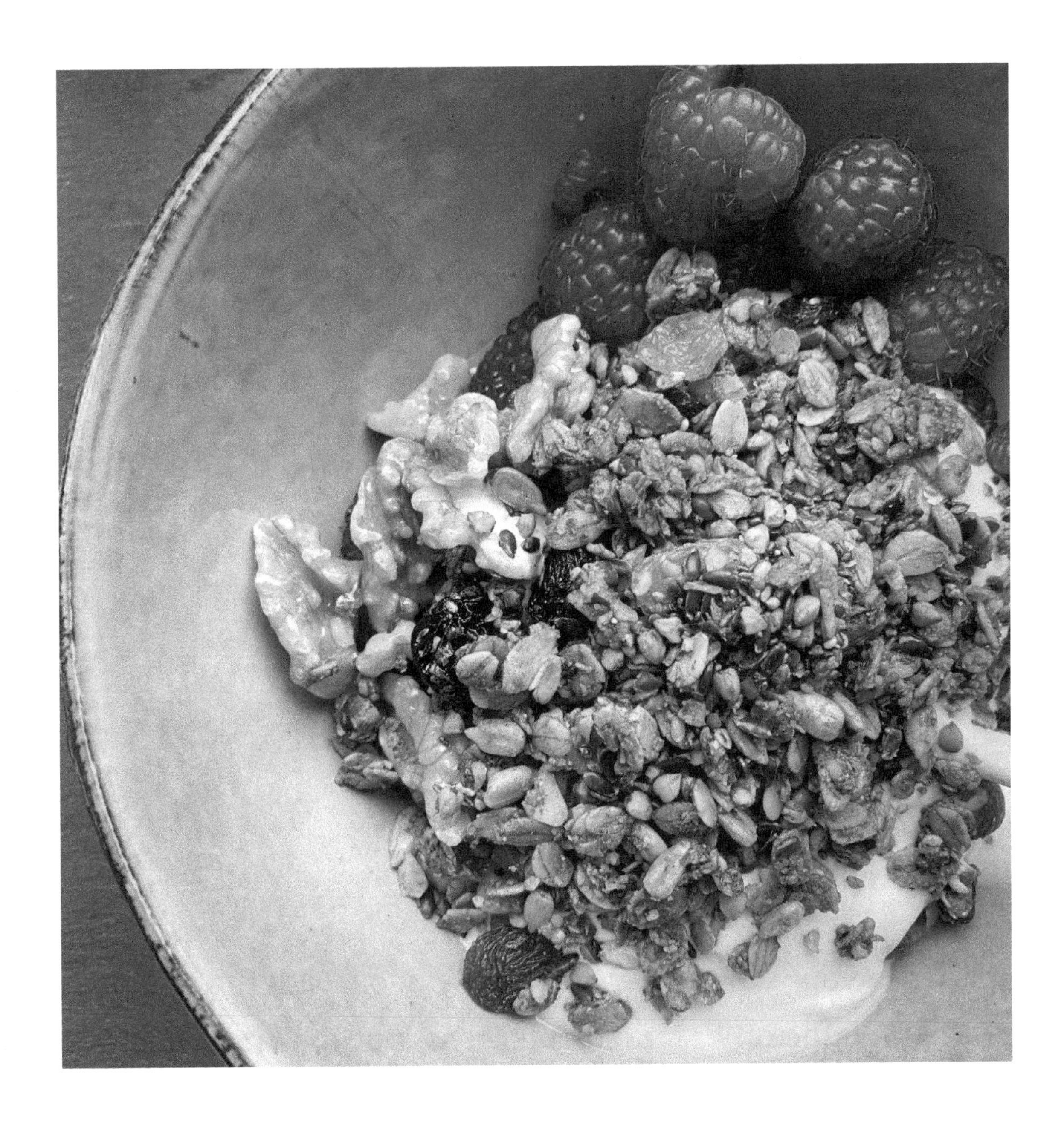

Preparation time: 10 minutes

Cooking time: 4 hours

Servings: 2

Ingredients:

- ½ cup granola
- ¼ cup coconut cream
- 2 tablespoons brown sugar
- 2 tablespoons cashew butter
- 1 teaspoon cinnamon powder
- ½ teaspoon nutmeg, ground

Directions:

1. In your slow cooker, mix the granola with the cream, sugar and the other ingredients, toss, put the lid on and cook on Low for 4 hours.
2. Divide into bowls and serve for breakfast.

Nutrition: calories 218, fat 6, fiber 9, carbs 17, protein 6

Cinnamon Quinoa

Preparation time: 10 minutes

Cooking time: 4 hours

Servings: 4

Ingredients:

- 1 cup quinoa
- 2 cups milk
- 2 cups water
- ¼ cup stevia
- 1 teaspoon cinnamon powder
- 1 teaspoon vanilla extract

Directions:

1. In your Slow cooker, mix quinoa with milk, water, stevia, cinnamon and vanilla, stir, cover, cook on Low for 3 hours and 30 minutes, stir, cook for 30 minutes more, divide into bowls and serve for breakfast.

Nutrition: calories 172, fat 4, fiber 3, carbs 8, protein 2

Squash Bowls

Preparation time: 10 minutes

Cooking time: 6 hours

Servings: 2

Ingredients:

- 2 tablespoons walnuts, chopped
- 2 cups squash, peeled and cubed
- ½ cup coconut cream
- ½ teaspoon cinnamon powder
- ½ tablespoon sugar

Directions:

1. In your slow cooker, mix the squash with the nuts and the other ingredients, toss, put the lid on and cook on Low for 6 hours.

2. Divide into bowls and serve.

Nutrition: calories 140, fat 1, fiber 2, carbs 2, protein 5

Quinoa and Apricots

Preparation time: 10 minutes

Cooking time: 10 hours

Servings: 6

Ingredients:

- ¾ cup quinoa
- ¾ cup steel cut oats
- 2 tablespoons honey
- 1 cup apricots, chopped
- 6 cups water
- 1 teaspoon vanilla extract
- ¾ cup hazelnuts, chopped

Directions:

1. In your Slow cooker, mix quinoa with oats honey, apricots, water, vanilla and hazelnuts, stir, cover and cook on Low for 10 hours.

2. Stir quinoa mix again, divide into bowls and serve for breakfast.

Nutrition: calories 200, fat 3, fiber 5, carbs 8, protein 6

Lamb and Eggs Mix

Preparation time: 10 minutes

Cooking time: 6 hours

Servings: 2

Ingredients:

- 1 pound lamb meat, ground
- 4 eggs, whisked
- 1 tablespoon basil, chopped
- ½ teaspoon cumin powder
- 1 tablespoon chili powder
- 1 red onion, chopped
- 1 tablespoon olive oil
- A pinch of salt and black pepper

Directions:

1. Grease the slow cooker with the oil and mix the lamb with the eggs, basil and the other ingredients inside.

2. Toss, put the lid on, cook on Low for 6 hours, divide into bowls and serve for breakfast.

Nutrition: calories 220, fat 2, fiber 2, carbs 6, protein 2

Blueberry Quinoa Oatmeal

Preparation time: 10 minutes

Cooking time: 8 hours

Servings: 4

Ingredients:

- ½ cup quinoa
- 1 cup steel cut oats
- 1 teaspoon vanilla extract
- 5 cups water
- Zest of 1 lemon, grated
- 1 teaspoon vanilla extract
- 2 tablespoons flaxseed
- 1 tablespoon butter, melted

- 3 tablespoons maple syrup
- 1 cup blueberries

Directions:

1. In your Slow cooker, mix butter with quinoa, water, oats, vanilla, lemon zest, flaxseed, maple syrup and blueberries, stir, cover and cook on Low for 8 hours.
2. Divide into bowls and serve for breakfast.

Nutrition: calories 189, fat 5, fiber 5, carbs 20, protein 5

Lunch Roast

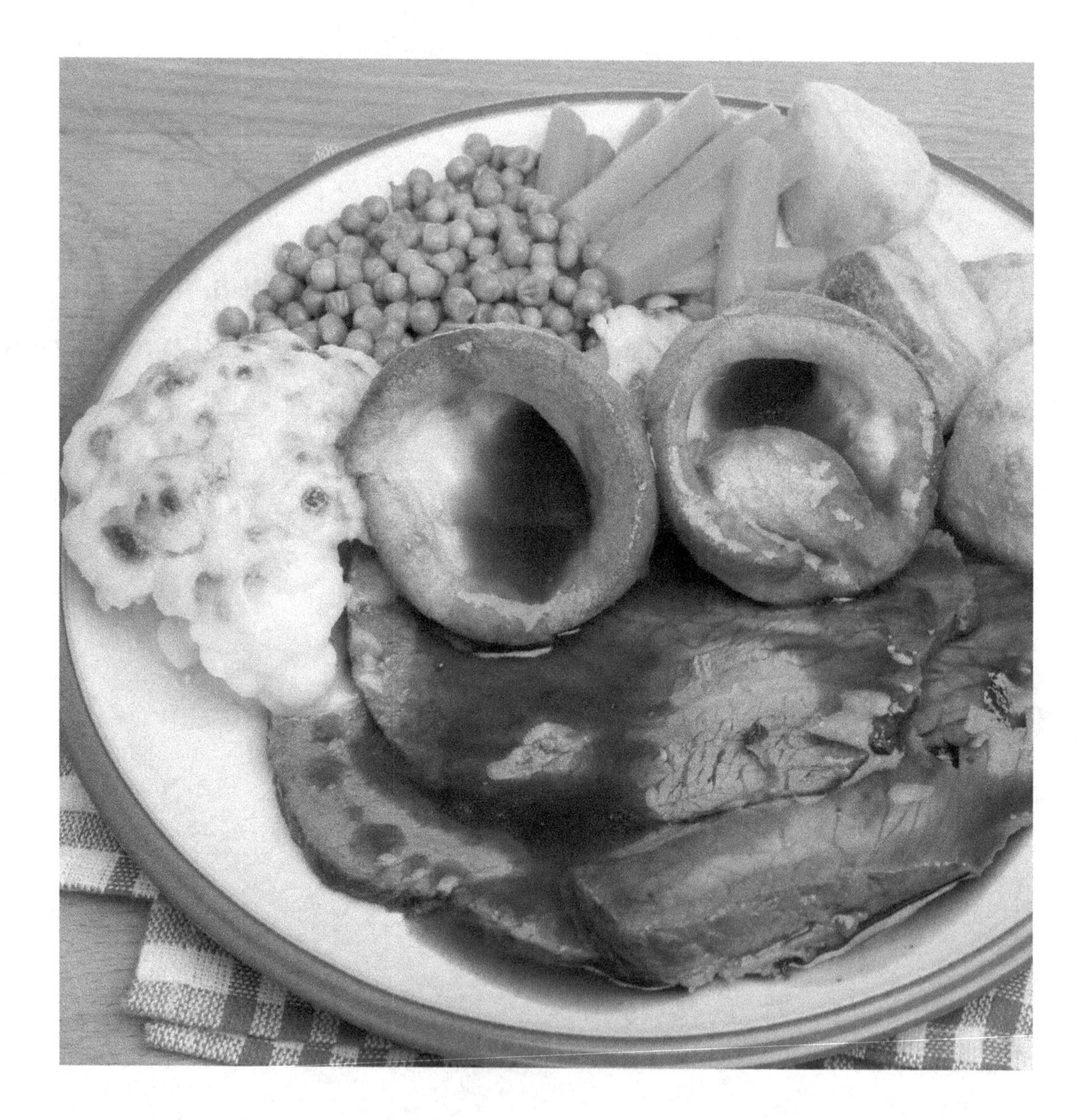

Preparation time: 10 minutes

Cooking time: 8 hours

Servings: 8

Ingredients:

- 2 pounds beef chuck roast
- Salt and black pepper to the taste
- 1 yellow onion, chopped
- 2 teaspoons olive oil
- 8 ounces tomato sauce
- ¼ cup lemon juice
- ¼ cup water
- ¼ cup ketchup
- ¼ cup apple cider vinegar
- 1 tablespoons Worcestershire sauce
- 2 tablespoons brown sugar
- ½ teaspoon mustard powder
- ½ teaspoons paprika

Directions:

1. In your Slow cooker, mix beef with salt, pepper, onion oil, tomato sauce, lemon juice, water, ketchup, vinegar, Worcestershire sauce, sugar, mustard and paprika, toss well, cover and cook on Low for 8 hours.

2. Slice roast, divide between plates, drizzle cooking sauce all over and serve for lunch.

Nutrition: calories 243, fat 12, fiber 2, carbs 10, protein 23

Sesame Salmon Bowls

Preparation time: 10 minutes

Cooking time: 3 hours

Servings: 2

Ingredients:

- 2 salmon fillets, boneless and roughly cubed
- 1 cup cherry tomatoes, halved
- 3 spring onions, chopped
- 1 cup baby spinach
- ½ cup chicken stock
- Salt and black pepper to the taste
- 2 tablespoons balsamic vinegar
- 2 tablespoons lemon juice

- 1 teaspoon sesame seeds

Directions:

1. In your slow cooker, mix the salmon with the cherry tomatoes, spring onions and the other ingredients, toss gently, put the lid on and cook on Low for 3 hours.

2. Divide everything into bowls and serve.

Nutrition: calories 230, fat 4, fiber 2, carbs 7, protein 6

Fajitas

Preparation time: 10 minutes

Cooking time: 3 hours

Servings: 8

Ingredients:

- 1 and ½ pounds beef sirloin, cut into thin strips
- 2 tablespoons lemon juice
- 2 tablespoons olive oil
- 1 garlic clove, minced
- 1 and ½ teaspoon cumin, ground
- Salt and black pepper to the taste
- ½ teaspoon chili powder

- A pinch of red pepper flakes, crushed
- 1 red bell pepper, cut into thin strips
- 1 yellow onion, cut into thin strips
- 8 mini tortillas

Directions:

1. Heat up a pan with the oil over medium-high heat, add beef strips, brown them for a few minutes and transfer to your Slow cooker.
2. Add lemon juice, garlic, cumin, salt, pepper, chili powder and pepper flakes to the slow cooker as well, cover and cook on High for 2 hours.
3. Add bell pepper and onion, stir and cook on High for 1 more hour.
4. Divide beef mix between your mini tortillas and serve for lunch.

Nutrition: calories 220, fat 9, fiber 2, carbs 14, protein 20

Shrimp Stew

Preparation time: 10 minutes

Cooking time: 3 hours

Servings: 2

Ingredients:

- 1 garlic clove, minced
- 1 red onion, chopped
- 1 cup canned tomatoes, crushed
- 1 cup veggie stock
- ½ teaspoon turmeric powder
- 1 pound shrimp, peeled and deveined
- ½ teaspoon coriander, ground
- ½ teaspoon thyme, dried

- ½ teaspoon basil, dried
- A pinch of salt and black pepper
- A pinch of red pepper flakes

Directions:

1. In your slow cooker, mix the onion with the garlic, shrimp and the other ingredients, toss, put the lid on and cook on High for 3 hours.
2. Divide the stew into bowls and serve.

Nutrition: calories 313, fat 4.2, fiber 2.5, carbs 13.2, protein 53.3

Teriyaki Pork

Preparation time: 10 minutes

Cooking time: 7 hours

Servings: 8

Ingredients:

- 2 tablespoons sugar
- 2 tablespoons soy sauce
- ¾ cup apple juice
- 1 teaspoon ginger powder
- 1 tablespoon white vinegar
- Salt and black pepper to the taste
- ¼ teaspoon garlic powder
- 3 pounds pork loin roast, halved

- 7 teaspoons cornstarch
- 3 tablespoons water

Directions:

1. In your Slow cooker, mix apple juice with sugar, soy sauce, vinegar, ginger, garlic powder, salt, pepper and pork loin, toss well, cover and cook on Low for 7 hours.
2. Transfer cooking juices to a small pan, heat up over medium-high heat, add cornstarch mixed with water, stir well, cook for 2 minutes until it thickens and take off heat.
3. Slice roast, divide between plates, drizzle sauce all over and serve for lunch.

Nutrition: calories 247, fat 8, fiber 1, carbs 9, protein 33

Garlic Shrimp and Spinach

Preparation time: 10 minutes

Cooking time: 2 hours

Servings: 2

Ingredients:

- 1 pound shrimp, peeled and deveined
- 1 cup baby spinach
- ½ teaspoon sweet paprika
- ½ cup chicken stock
- 1 garlic clove, minced
- 2 jalapeno peppers, chopped
- Cooking spray
- 1 teaspoon coriander, ground

- ½ teaspoon rosemary, dried
- A pinch of sea salt and black pepper

Directions:

1. Grease the slow cooker with the oil, add the shrimp, spinach and the other ingredients, toss, put the lid on and cook on High for 2 hours.
2. Divide everything between plates and serve for lunch.

Nutrition: calories 200, fat 4, fiber 6, carbs 16, protein 4

Beef Stew

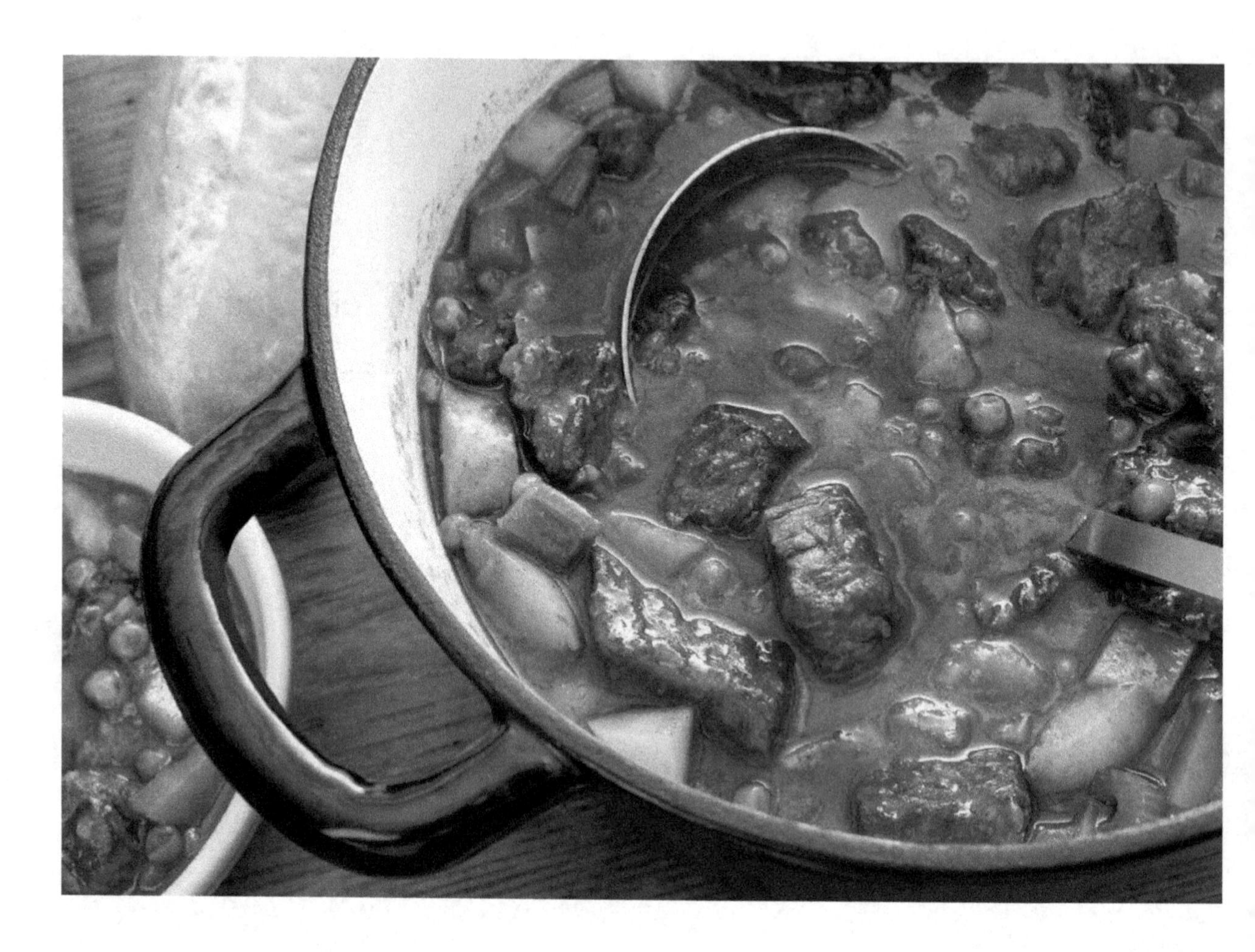

Preparation time: 10 minutes

Cooking time: 7 hours and 30 minutes

Servings: 5

Ingredients:

- 2 potatoes, peeled and cubed
- 1 pound beef stew meat, cubed
- 11 ounces tomato juice
- 14 ounces beef stock
- 2 celery ribs, chopped
- 2 carrots, chopped
- 3 bay leaves
- 1 yellow onion, chopped
- Salt and black pepper to the taste
- ½ teaspoon chili powder
- ½ teaspoon thyme, dried
- 1 tablespoon water
- 2 tablespoons cornstarch
- ½ cup peas
- ½ cup corn

Directions:

1. In your Slow cooker, mix potatoes with beef, tomato juice, stock, ribs, carrots, bay leaves, onion, salt, pepper, chili powder and thyme, stir, cover and cook on Low for 7 hours.

2. Add cornstarch mixed with water, peas and corn, stir, cover and cook on Low for 30 minutes more.

3. Divide into bowls and serve for lunch.

Nutrition: calories 273, fat 7, fiber 6, carbs 30, protein 22

Ginger Salmon

Preparation time: 10 minutes

Cooking time: 3 hours

Servings: 2

Ingredients:

- 2 salmon fillets, boneless
- 1 tablespoon olive oil
- 1 tablespoon balsamic vinegar
- 1 tablespoon ginger, grated
- A pinch of nutmeg, ground
- A pinch of cloves, ground
- A pinch of salt and black pepper
- 1 teaspoon onion powder

- ½ teaspoon cayenne pepper
- ¼ cup chicken stock

Directions:

1. Grease the slow cooker with the oil and arrange the salmon fillets inside.
2. Add the vinegar, ginger and the other ingredients, rub gently, put the lid on and cook on Low for 3 hours.
3. Divide the fish between plates and serve with a side salad for lunch.

Nutrition: calories 315, fat 18.4, fiber 0.6, carbs 3.6, protein 35.1

Apple and Onion Lunch Roast

Preparation time: 10 minutes

Cooking time: 5 hours

Servings: 8

Ingredients:

- 1 beef sirloin roast, halved
- Salt and black pepper to the taste
- 1 cup water
- ½ teaspoon soy sauce
- 1 apple, cored and quartered
- ¼ teaspoon garlic powder
- ½ teaspoon Worcestershire sauce
- 1 yellow onion, cut into medium wedges

- 2 tablespoons water
- 2 tablespoons cornstarch
- 1/8 teaspoon browning sauce
- Cooking spray

Directions:

1. Grease a pan with the cooking spray, heat it up over medium-high heat, add roast, brown it for a few minutes on each side and transfer to your Slow cooker.
2. Add salt, pepper, soy sauce, garlic powder, Worcestershire sauce, onion and apple, cover and cook on Low for 6 hours.
3. Transfer cooking juices from the slow cooker to a pan, heat it up over medium heat, add cornstarch, water and browning sauce, stir well, cook for a few minutes and take off heat.
4. Slice roast, divide between plates, drizzle sauce all over and serve for lunch.

Nutrition: calories 242, fat 8, fiber 1, carbs 8, protein 34

Creamy Cod Stew

Preparation time: 10 minutes

Cooking time: 3 hours

Servings: 2

Ingredients:

- ½ pound cod fillets, boneless and cubed
- 2 spring onions, chopped
- ¼ cup heavy cream
- 1 carrot, sliced
- 1 zucchini, cubed
- 1 tomato, cubed
- 1 cup chicken stock
- 1 tablespoon olive oil

- 1 green bell pepper, chopped
- 1 tablespoon chives, chopped
- A pinch of salt and black pepper

Directions:

1. In your slow cooker, combine the fish with the spring onions, carrot and the other ingredients except the cream, toss gently, put the lid on and cook on High for 2 hours and 30 minutes.
2. Add the cream, toss gently, put the lid back on, cook the stew on Low for 30 minutes more, divide into bowls and serve.

Nutrition: calories 175, fat 13.3, fiber 3.4, carbs 14, protein 3.3

Stuffed Peppers

Preparation time: 10 minutes

Cooking time: 4 hours

Servings: 4

Ingredients:

- 15 ounces canned black beans, drained
- 4 sweet red peppers, tops and seeds discarded
- 1 cup pepper jack cheese, shredded
- 1 yellow onion, chopped
- ¾ cup salsa
- ½ cup corn
- 1/3 cup white rice
- ½ teaspoon cumin, ground

- 1 and ½ teaspoons chili powder

Directions:

1. In a bowl, mix black beans with cheese, salsa, onion, corn, rice, cumin and chili powder and stir well.
2. Stuff peppers with this mix, place them in your Slow cooker, cover and cook on Low for 4 hours.
3. Divide between plates and serve them for lunch.

Nutrition: calories 317, fat 10, fiber 8, carbs 43, protein 12

Sweet Potato and Clam Chowder

Preparation time: 10 minutes

Cooking time: 3 hours and 30 minutes

Servings: 2

Ingredients:

- 1 small yellow onion, chopped
- 1 carrot, chopped
- 1 red bell pepper, cubed
- 6 ounces canned clams, chopped
- 1 sweet potato, chopped
- 2 cups chicken stock
- ½ cup coconut milk
- 1 teaspoon Worcestershire sauce

Directions:

1. In your slow cooker, mix the onion with the carrot, clams and the other ingredients, toss, put the lid on and cook on High for 3 hours.

2. Divide the chowder into bowls and serve for lunch.

Nutrition: calories 288, fat 15.3, fiber 5.9, carbs 36.4, protein 5

Beans and Pumpkin Chili

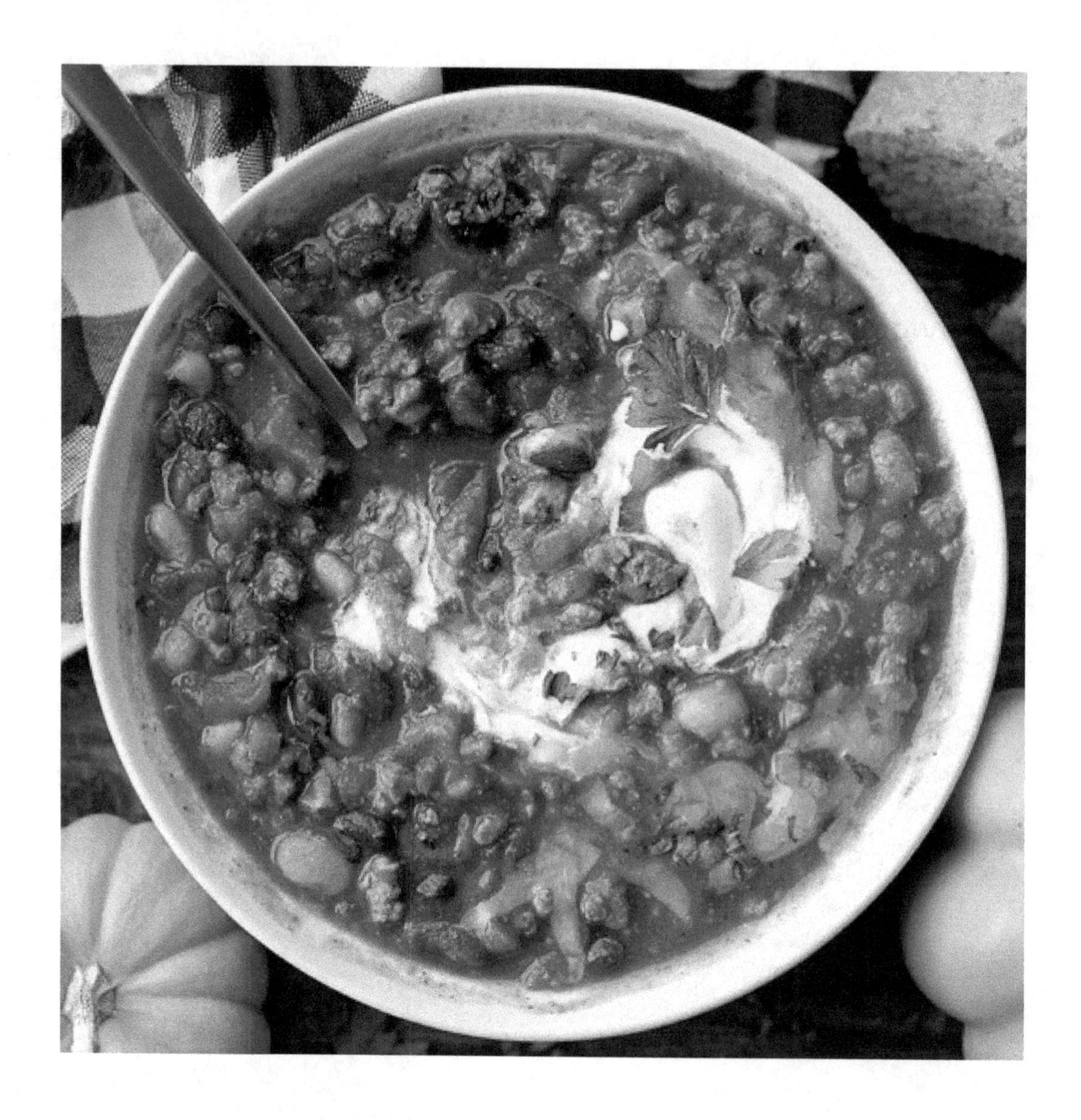

Preparation time: 10 minutes

Cooking time: 4 hours

Servings: 10

Ingredients:

- 1 yellow bell pepper, chopped
- 1 yellow onion, chopped
- 3 garlic cloves, minced
- 2 tablespoons olive oil
- 3 cups chicken stock
- 30 ounces canned black beans, drained
- 14 ounces pumpkin, cubed
- 2 and ½ cups turkey meat, cooked and cubed
- 2 teaspoons parsley, dried
- 1 and ½ teaspoon oregano, dried
- 2 teaspoons chili powder
- 1 and ½ teaspoon cumin, ground
- Salt and black pepper to the taste

Directions:

1. Heat up a pan with the oil over medium-high heat, add bell pepper, onion and garlic, stir, cook for a few minutes and transfer to your Slow cooker.

2. Add stock, beans, pumpkin, turkey, parsley, oregano, chili powder, cumin, salt and pepper, stir, cover and cook on Low for 4 hours.

3. Divide into bowls and serve right away for lunch.

Nutrition: calories 200, fat 5, fiber 7, carbs 20, protein 15

Maple Chicken Mix

Preparation time: 10 minutes

Cooking time: 6 hours

Servings: 2

Ingredients:

- 2 spring onions, chopped
- 1 pound chicken breast, skinless and boneless
- 2 garlic cloves, minced
- 1 tablespoon maple syrup
- A pinch of salt and black pepper
- ½ cup chicken stock
- ½ cup tomato sauce
- 1 tablespoon chives, chopped

- 1 teaspoon basil, dried

Directions:

1. In your slow cooker mix the chicken with the garlic, maple syrup and the other ingredients, toss, put the lid on and cook on Low for 6 hours.
2. Divide the mix between plates and serve for lunch.

Nutrition: calories 200, fat 3, fiber 3, carbs 17, protein 6

Chicken and Peppers Mix

Preparation time: 10 minutes

Cooking time: 4 hours

Servings: 6

Ingredients:

- 24 ounces tomato sauce
- ¼ cup parmesan, grated
- 1 yellow onion, chopped
- 2 garlic cloves, minced
- 1 teaspoon basil, dried
- 1 teaspoon oregano, dried
- Salt and black pepper to the taste
- 6 chicken breast halves, skinless and boneless

- ½ green bell pepper, chopped
- ½ yellow bell pepper, chopped
- ½ red bell pepper, chopped

Directions:

1. In your Slow cooker, mix tomato sauce with parmesan, onion, garlic, basil, oregano, salt, pepper, chicken, green bell pepper, yellow bell pepper and red bell pepper, toss, cover and cook on Low for 4 hours.
2. Divide between plates and serve for lunch.

Nutrition: calories 221, fat 6, fiber 3, carbs 16, protein 26

Salsa Chicken

Preparation time: 10 minutes

Cooking time: 8 hours

Servings: 2

Ingredients:

- 7 ounces mild salsa
- 1 pound chicken breast, skinless, boneless and cubed
- 1 small yellow onion, chopped
- ½ teaspoon coriander, ground
- ½ teaspoon rosemary, dried
- 1 green bell pepper, chopped
- Cooking spray
- 1 tablespoon cilantro, chopped

- 1 red bell pepper, chopped
- 1 tablespoon chili powder

Directions:

1. Grease the slow cooker with the cooking spray and mix the chicken with the salsa, onion and the other ingredients inside.
2. Put the lid on, cook on Low for 8 hours, divide into bowls and serve for lunch.

Nutrition: calories 240, fat 3, fiber 7, carbs 17, protein 8

Chicken Tacos

Preparation time: 10 minutes

Cooking time: 5 hours

Servings: 16

Ingredients:

- 2 mangos, peeled and chopped
- 2 tomatoes, chopped
- 1 and ½ cups pineapple chunks
- 1 red onion, chopped
- 2 small green bell peppers, chopped
- 1 tablespoon lime juice
- 2 green onions, chopped

- 1 teaspoon sugar
- 4 pounds chicken breast halves, skinless
- Salt and black pepper to the taste
- 32 taco shells, warm
- ¼ cup cilantro, chopped
- ¼ cup brown sugar

Directions:

1. In a bowl, mix mango with pineapple, red onion, tomatoes, bell peppers, green onions and lime juice and toss.
2. Put chicken in your Slow cooker, add salt, pepper and sugar and toss.
3. Add mango mix, cover and cook on Low for 5 hours.
4. Transfer chicken to a cutting board, cool it down, discard bones and shred meat.
5. Divide meat and mango mix between taco shells and serve them for lunch.

Nutrition: calories 246, fat 7, fiber 2, carbs 25, protein 21

Turkey and Mushrooms

Preparation time: 10 minutes

Cooking time: 7 hours and 10 minutes

Servings: 2

Ingredients:

- 1 red onion, sliced
- 2 garlic cloves, minced
- 1 pound turkey breast, skinless, boneless and cubed
- 1 tablespoon olive oil
- 1 teaspoon oregano, dried
- 1 teaspoon basil, dried
- A pinch of red pepper flakes
- 1 cup mushrooms, sliced

- ¼ cup chicken stock
- ½ cup canned tomatoes, chopped
- A pinch of salt and black pepper

Directions:

1. Heat up a pan with the oil over medium-high heat, add the onion , garlic and the meat, brown for 10 minutes and transfer to the slow cooker.
2. Add the oregano, basil and the other ingredients, toss, put the lid on and cook on Low for 7 hours.
3. Divide into bowls and serve for lunch.

Nutrition: calories 240, fat 4, fiber 6, carbs 18, protein 10

Orange Beef Dish

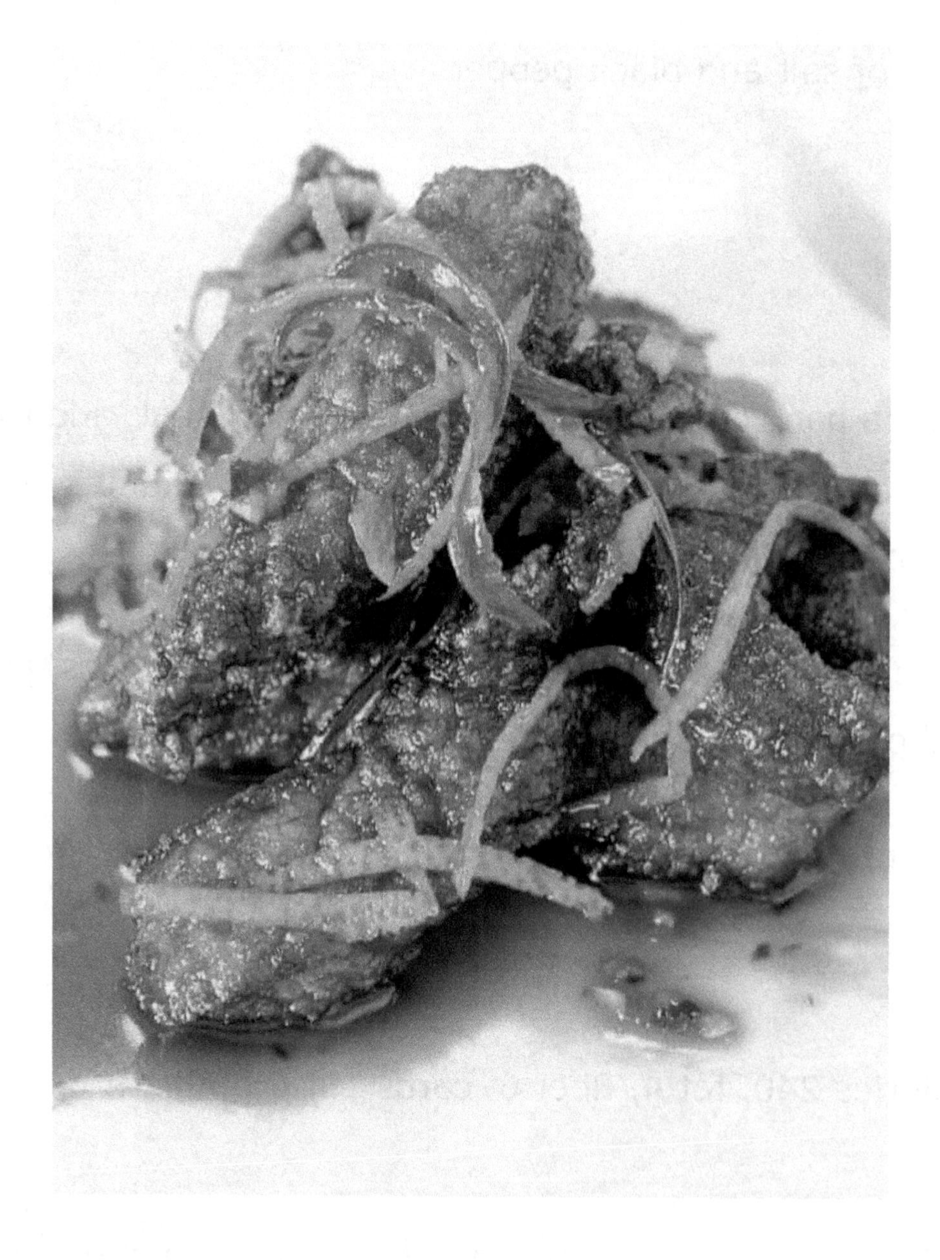

Preparation time: 10 minutes

Cooking time: 5 hours

Servings: 5

Ingredients:

- 1 pound beef sirloin steak, cut into medium strips
- 2 and ½ cups shiitake mushrooms, sliced
- 1 yellow onion, cut into medium wedges
- 3 red hot chilies, dried
- ¼ cup brown sugar
- ¼ cup orange juice
- ¼ cup soy sauce
- 2 tablespoons cider vinegar
- 1 tablespoon cornstarch
- 1 tablespoon ginger, grated
- 1 tablespoon sesame oil
- 1 cup snow peas

- 2 garlic cloves, minced
- 1 tablespoon orange zest, grated

Directions:

1. In your Slow cooker, mix steak strips with mushrooms, onion, chilies, sugar, orange juice, soy sauce, vinegar, cornstarch, ginger, oil, garlic and orange zest, toss, cover and cook on Low for 4 hours and 30 minutes.
2. Add snow peas, cover, cook on Low for 30 minutes more, divide between plates and serve.

Nutrition: calories 310, fat 7, fiber 4, carbs 26, protein 33

Indian Chicken and Tomato Mix

Preparation time: 10 minutes

Cooking time: 6 hours

Servings: 2

Ingredients:

- 1 cup cherry tomatoes, halved
- 1 pound chicken breast, skinless, boneless and cubed
- 1 red onion, sliced
- 1 tablespoons garam masala
- 1 garlic clove, minced
- ½ small yellow onion, chopped
- ½ teaspoon ginger powder
- A pinch of salt and cayenne pepper

- ½ teaspoon sweet paprika
- 2 tablespoons chives, chopped

Directions:

1. In your slow cooker, mix the chicken with the tomatoes, onion and the other ingredients, toss, put the lid on and cook on Low for 6 hours.
2. Divide into bowls and serve right away.

Nutrition: calories 259, fat 3, fiber 7, carbs 17, protein 14

Chicken with Couscous

Preparation time: 10 minutes

Cooking time: 3 hours

Servings: 6

Ingredients:

- 2 sweet potatoes, peeled and cubed
- 1 sweet red peppers, chopped
- 1 and ½ pounds chicken breasts, skinless and boneless
- 13 ounces canned stewed tomatoes
- Salt and black pepper to the taste
- ¼ cup raisins
- ¼ teaspoon cinnamon powder
- ¼ teaspoon cumin, ground

For the couscous:

- 1 cup whole wheat couscous
- 1 cup water
- Salt to the taste

Directions:

1. In your Slow cooker, mix potatoes with red peppers, chicken, tomatoes, salt, pepper, raisins, cinnamon and cumin, toss, cover, cook on Low for 3 hours and shred meat using 2 forks.
2. Meanwhile, heat up a pan with the water over medium-high heat, add salt, bring water to a boil, add couscous, stir, leave aside covered for 10 minutes and fluff with a fork.
3. Divide chicken mix between plates, add couscous on the side and serve.

Nutrition: calories 351, fat 4, fiber 7, carbs 45, protein 30

Turkey and Figs

Preparation time: 10 minutes

Cooking time: 8 hours

Servings: 2

Ingredients:

- 1 pound turkey breast, boneless, skinless and sliced
- ½ cup black figs, halved
- 1 red onion, sliced
- ½ cup tomato sauce
- ½ teaspoon onion powder
- ¼ teaspoon garlic powder
- 1 tablespoon basil, chopped
- ½ teaspoon chili powder

- ¼ cup white wine
- ½ teaspoon thyme, dried
- ¼ teaspoon sage, dried
- ½ teaspoon paprika, dried
- A pinch of salt and black pepper

Directions:

1. In your slow cooker, mix the turkey breast with the figs, onion and the other ingredients, toss, put the lid on and cook on Low for 8 hours.
2. Divide between plates and serve.

Nutrition: calories 220, fat 5, fiber 8, carbs 18, protein 15

Pork Stew

Preparation time: 10 minutes

Cooking time: 5 hours

Servings: 8

Ingredients:

- 2 pork tenderloins, cubed
- Salt and black pepper to the taste
- 2 carrots, sliced
- 1 yellow onion, chopped
- 2 celery ribs, chopped
- 2 tablespoons tomato paste
- 3 cups beef stock
- 1/3 cup plums, dried, pitted and chopped

- 1 rosemary spring
- 1 thyme spring
- 2 bay leaves
- 4 garlic cloves, minced
- 1/3 cup green olives, pitted and sliced
- 1 tablespoon parsley, chopped

Directions:

1. In your Slow cooker, mix pork with salt, pepper, carrots, onion, celery, tomato paste, stock, plums, rosemary, thyme, bay leaves, garlic, olives and parsley, cover and cook on Low for 5 hours.
2. Discard thyme, rosemary and bay leaves, divide stew into bowls and serve for lunch.

Nutrition: calories 200, fat 4, fiber 2, carbs 8, protein 23

Turkey and Walnuts

Preparation time: 10 minutes

Cooking time: 8 hours

Servings: 2

Ingredients:

- 1 pound turkey breast, skinless, boneless and sliced
- ½ cup scallions, chopped
- 2 tablespoons walnuts, chopped
- 1 tablespoon lemon juice
- ¼ cup veggie stock
- ½ teaspoon chili powder
- 1 tablespoon olive oil
- 1 tablespoon rosemary, chopped

- Salt and black pepper to the taste

Directions:

1. In your slow cooker, mix the turkey with the scallions, walnuts and the other ingredients, toss, put the lid on and cook on Low for 8 hours.
2. Divide everything between plates and serve.

Nutrition: calories 264, fat 4, fiber 6, carbs 15, protein 15

Seafood Stew

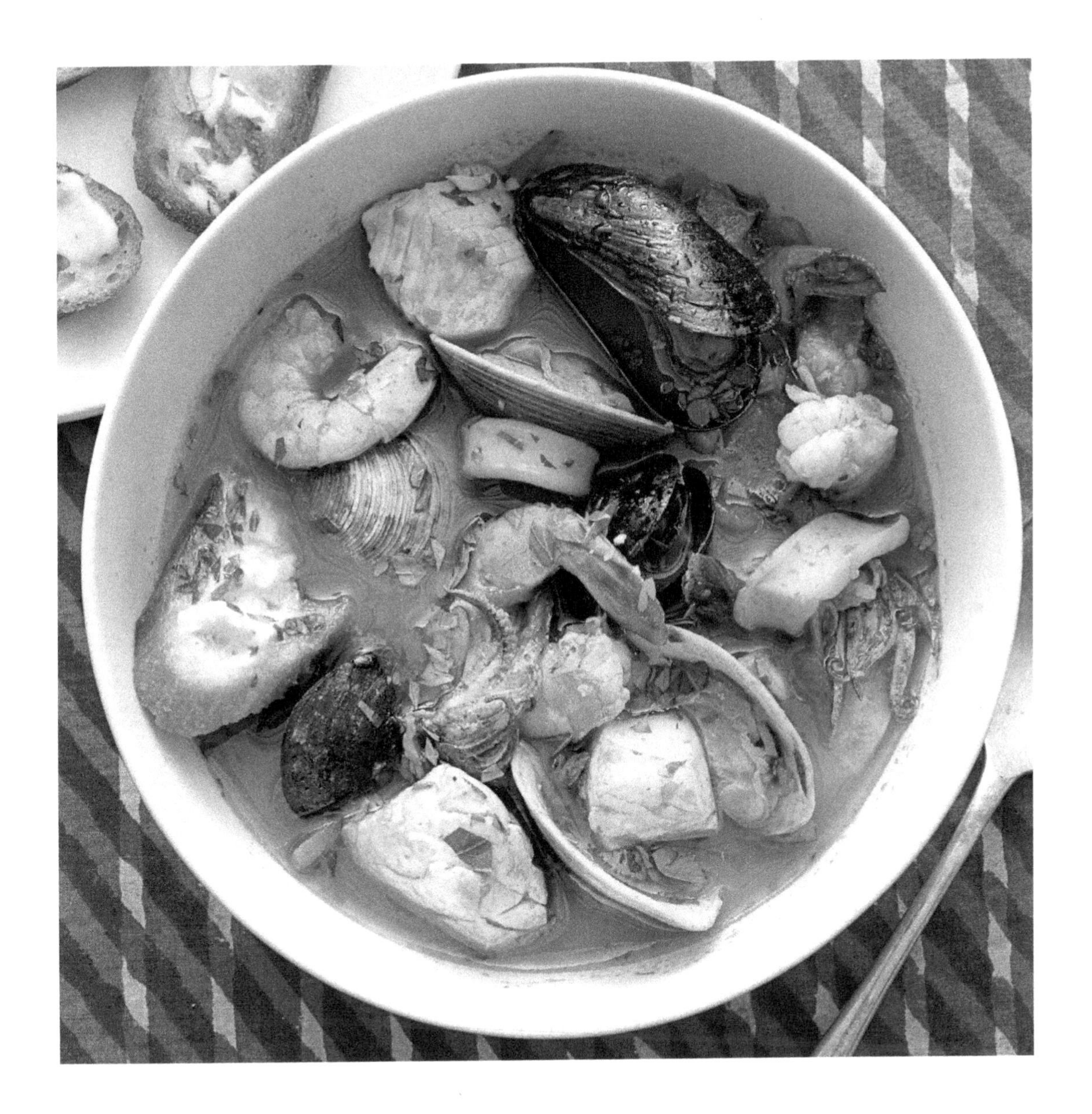

Preparation time: 10 minutes

Cooking time: 4 hours and 30 minutes

Servings: 8

Ingredients:

- 8 ounces clam juice
- 2 yellow onions, chopped
- 28 ounces canned tomatoes, chopped
- 6 ounces tomato paste
- 3 celery ribs, chopped
- ½ cup white wine
- 1 tablespoon red vinegar
- 5 garlic cloves, minced
- 1 tablespoon olive oil
- 1 teaspoon Italian seasoning
- 1 bay leaf
- 1 pound haddock fillets, boneless and cut into medium pieces

- ½ teaspoon sugar
- 1 pound shrimp, peeled and deveined
- 6 ounces crabmeat
- 6 ounces canned clams
- 2 tablespoons parsley, chopped

Directions:

1. In your Slow cooker, mix tomatoes with onions, clam juice, tomato paste, celery, wine, vinegar, garlic, oil, seasoning, sugar and bay leaf, stir, cover and cook on Low for 4 hours.
2. Add shrimp, haddock, crabmeat and clams, cover, cook on Low for 30 minutes more, divide into bowls and serve with parsley sprinkled on top.

Nutrition: calories 205, fat 4, fiber 4, carbs 14, protein 27

Slow Cooked Thyme Chicken

Preparation time: 10 minutes

Cooking time: 7 hours

Servings: 2

Ingredients:

- 1 pound chicken legs
- 1 tablespoon thyme, chopped
- 2 garlic cloves, minced
- ½ cup chicken stock
- 1 carrot, chopped
- ½ yellow onion, chopped
- A pinch of salt and white pepper
- Juice of ½ lemon

Directions:

1. In your slow cooker, mix the chicken legs with the thyme, garlic and the other ingredients, toss, put the lid on and cook on Low for 7 hours.

2. Divide between plates and serve.

Nutrition: calories 320, fat 4, fiber 7, carbs 16, protein 6

Conclusion

Did you indulge in attempting these brand-new and also delicious recipes?
regrettably we have come to the end of this slow cooker recipe book, I really want it has actually been to your liking. to improve your health and wellness and wellness we would certainly like to recommend you to incorporate workout as well as additionally a vibrant way of living together with adhere to these superb meals, so regarding emphasize the enhancements. we will definitely be back soon with other significantly interesting vegan dishes, a big hug, see you soon.

CPSIA information can be obtained
at www.ICGtesting.com
Printed in the USA
BVHW051943250521
608097BV00003B/745